Weight Loss Guide

5 Tips to Lose  Weight

By

Dr. Hannah collins

# Table of Contents

# Table of Contents

# Introduction

## The Journey to a Healthier You

Embarking on the path to a healthier lifestyle entails more than just a desire to lose weight; it also entails developing habits that lead to long-term health. This path addresses physical, mental, and emotional health in order to improve overall quality of life. The important components are:

1. Balanced Diet: A well-rounded diet that includes fruits, vegetables, lean proteins, whole grains, and healthy fats.
2. Regular Exercise: Performing physical activities that improve cardiovascular health, strength, flexibility, and endurance.
3. Mental Health: Managing stress, getting enough sleep, and receiving emotional assistance as needed.
4. Consistency and Patience: Recognize that long-term health changes require continual commitment and patience.

Understanding Weight Loss: Myths and Facts

Weight reduction is frequently surrounded by myths and misconceptions, which can stymie progress or lead to unhealthy habits. It's important to distinguish between myths and scientifically supported facts.

1. Myth: Rapid weight loss is the best strategy.
- Fact: Slow weight loss (1-2 pounds per week) is more sustainable and healthy. Rapid weight reduction can result in muscle loss, nutritional deficits, and other health complications.

2. Myth: Carbohydrates are unhealthy and should be avoided.
- Fact: Not all carbohydrates are equal. Whole grains, fruits, and vegetables contain critical nutrients and energy. Refined carbohydrates and sweets should be restricted.

3. Myth: Skipping meals can help you lose weight.

- Fact: Skipping meals can decrease metabolism, contribute to overeating later, and deplete the body of essential nutrients. Regular, balanced meals are essential.

4. Myth: Weight loss supplements are effective and safe.
- Fact: Most weight loss products lack strong proof of efficacy and may pose health hazards. Healthy food and regular exercise are still the safest and most effective strategies.

5. Myth: You can eliminate fat in certain regions.
- Fact: Spot reduction is impossible. Fat loss happens throughout the body as a result of genetics and lifestyle, rather than through specific activity.

Setting Realistic Goals.

Setting realistic objectives is an important step toward achieving and sustaining weight loss. Realistic objectives are specific, measurable, achievable, relevant, and time-bound (SMART).

1. Specific: Define what you intend to achieve. Instead of "I want to lose weight," say, "I want to lose 10 pounds."

2. Measurable: Make sure your aim is trackable and measurable. Use measures such as pounds lost, inches lowered, and body fat percentage.

3. Achievable: Set goals that are realistic for your existing lifestyle and finances. Consider your daily routine, physical abilities, and access to nutritious foods and exercise facilities.

4. Relevant: Your goals should be in line with your overall health aims and important to you. For example, if you have hypertension, you could try to lower your blood pressure by losing weight.

5. Time-bound: Create a schedule for reaching your objectives. Setting short-term goals, such as losing two pounds in the next month, might help you stay motivated and track your progress.

Focusing on these areas allows you to develop a long-term plan for a better living. To ensure long-term success in your health journey, you must first educate yourself, refute myths, and create sensible, attainable goals.

# Chapter 1

## Tip 1: Balanced Nutrition.

The Importance of a Balanced Diet.

A healthy diet is essential for good health and nutrition.it protects you against many chronic noncommunicable diseases. It ensures that your body receives the nutrients it requires to function properly, promotes development and repair, and aids in the prevention of chronic illnesses such as heart disease, diabetes, and obesity. A well-balanced diet often comprises a range of foods from all food groups, with adequate macronutrient (carbohydrates, proteins, and fats) and micronutrient (vitamins and minerals) ratios.

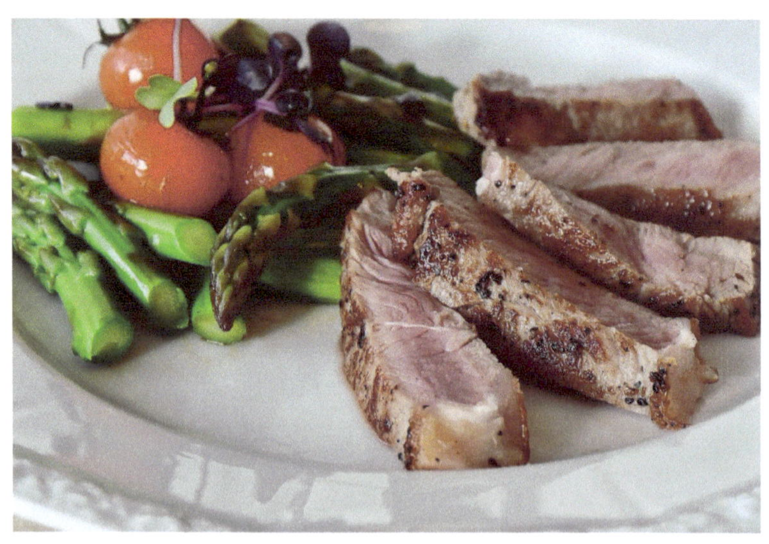

Macronutrients and micronutrients.

1) Macronutrients:

- Carbohydrates are the nutrients most frequently used as an energy source (containing

4 kcal per gram), as they are fast-acting and turn into energy as soon as they are ingested.
Foods that include it include cereals, fruits, vegetables, and legumes.

- Proteins are necessary for growth, tissue repair, and immunological function. Meat, fish, dairy products, beans, and nuts are all potential sources.

- Fats are essential for brain health, energy, and cell function. Avocados, almonds, seeds, and oily seafood all contain healthy fats.

2) Micronutrients:

- Vitamins: Organic substances needed in trace amounts for diverse human activities. Vitamin C (found in citrus fruits) is essential for immunological function, while vitamin D (found in fatty fish and fortified dairy products) promotes bone health.

- Minerals are inorganic elements that aid in activities like bone formation (calcium) and oxygen transfer (iron). Dairy products, green leafy vegetables, and meat are all potential sources.

Developing a Sustainable Meal Plan

A sustainable meal plan is realistic, fun, and long-lasting. It should include a wide variety of foods to avoid nutritional deficits and dietary boredom.

The key components are:
- Variety: Include items from each food group to get a wide range of nutrients.
- Moderation: Balance your intake of several food groups and avoid overconsumption of any one type of food.

- Flexibility: Allow for occasional indulgences while adapting to individual preferences and lifestyles.

Understanding Portion Control.

Portion control is vital for avoiding overeating and managing weight. It entails being aware of the amount of food ingested in one sitting. Practical tips include using smaller dishes to limit meal intake.
- Reading Labels: Understand the serving sizes and nutritional facts.
- Listen to your body: Eat when you're hungry, and quit when you're satisfied.

Sample Meal Plans and Recipes

Sample Meal Plan 1: - Breakfast: Greek yogurt with honey and mixed berries.
- Lunch: Grilled chicken salad with mixed veggies and a vinaigrette dressing.
- Snack: One handful of almonds.
- Dinner is baked salmon with quinoa and steamed broccoli.

Sample Meal Plan 2: - For breakfast, top oatmeal with banana slices and chia seeds.
- Lunch: Lentil soup and whole grain toast.
- Snack: Carrot sticks with hummus.
- Dinner is stir-fried tofu with mixed vegetables and brown rice.

Recipe for Quinoa Salad: - 1 cup cooked quinoa - 1 cup halved cherry tomatoes - 1 diced cucumber - 1/4 cup finely chopped red onion - 1/4 cup crumbled feta cheese.

- Add 2 tablespoons of olive oil and 1 tablespoon lemon juice.

- Season to taste with salt and pepper. - Instructions:

1. In a large bowl, combine the quinoa, cherry tomatoes, cucumber, red onion, and feta cheese.

2. In a small bowl, whisk together the olive oil, lemon juice, salt, and pepper.

3. Tossed salad with the dressing until well combined.

4. Serve chilled or warm.

These notes provide a thorough review of balanced nutrition, outlining its significance, the roles of various nutrients, how to develop a sustainable meal plan, the importance of portion control, and providing practical meal plans and recipes

# Chapter 2

## Tip 2:Regular Physical Activity

1. The Benefits of Exercise for Weight Loss
Regular physical activity is crucial for effective
weight management and overall health. Exercise
helps create a calorie deficit, meaning you burn
more calories than you consume, which is
essential for weight loss.

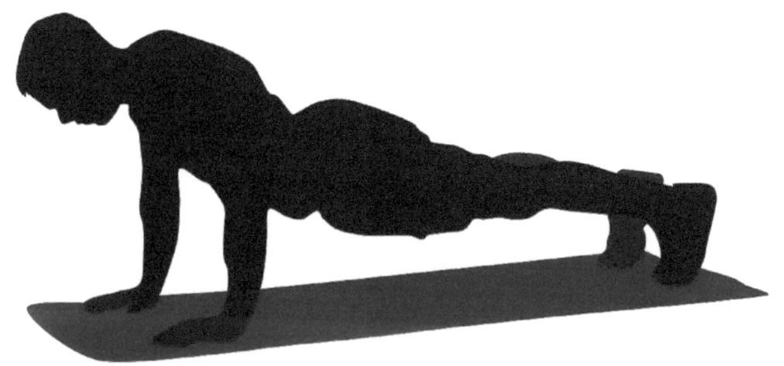

Key Points:

- Caloric Expenditure: Exercise increases the number of calories burned, aiding in weight loss by creating a calorie deficit.

- Metabolic Boost: Physical activity can boost your metabolism, helping you burn more calories even at rest.

- Preservation of Muscle Mass: Exercise, particularly strength training, helps preserve lean muscle mass during weight loss, which is important for maintaining a healthy metabolism.

- Enhanced Fat Burning: Regular exercise, especially high-intensity workouts, can enhance fat oxidation, helping you lose fat more efficiently.

- Improved Insulin Sensitivity: Exercise can improve insulin sensitivity, reducing the risk of type 2 diabetes and aiding in better weight management.

- Appetite Regulation: Regular physical activity can help regulate appetite and reduce overeating by influencing hunger hormones.

2. Types of Exercises: Cardiovascular, Strength Training, Flexibility A balanced exercise routine should include various types of exercises to

ensure comprehensive fitness and health benefits.

Key Points:
- Cardiovascular (Cardio) Exercise: - Examples: Running, cycling, swimming, brisk walking, dancing.
 - Benefits: Improves heart health, increases lung capacity, burns a high number of calories, and enhances endurance.
- Strength Training: - Examples: Weight lifting, bodyweight exercises (push-ups, squats), resistance band exercises.
- Benefits: Builds and preserves muscle mass, strengthens bones, increases metabolism, and improves overall body strength.
- Flexibility Training: - Examples: Stretching exercises, yoga, Pilates.

- Benefits: Enhances range of motion, reduces the risk of injury, alleviates muscle stiffness, and promotes relaxation.

3. Designing an Effective Workout Routine An effective workout routine is well-rounded, aligns with personal fitness goals, and includes a mix of cardio, strength, and flexibility exercises.

Key Points:
- Set fitness Goals: Identify what you want to achieve such as weight loss, muscle gain and improved endurance.
- Balanced Routine: Incorporate all three types of exercises: cardio for heart health and calorie burn, strength training for muscle building and metabolism boost, and flexibility exercises for range of motion and injury prevention.

- Frequency: Aim for at least 150 minutes of moderate-intensity cardio per week, two to three days of strength training, and daily flexibility exercises.
- Progressive Overload: Gradually increase the intensity, duration, and frequency of workouts to continue making progress.
- Rest and Recovery: Ensure adequate rest between workouts, especially strength training sessions, to allow muscle recovery and prevent overtraining.

4. Staying Motivated: Tips and Strategies
Staying motivated to exercise regularly can be challenging. Employing various strategies can help maintain consistency and enjoyment.

Key Points:

- Set dependable Goals: Start with simplest goals and gradually increase the difficulty as you progress.

 - Monitor Progress: Keep a workout journal or use fitness apps to track progress and celebrate milestones.

 - Find Enjoyable Activities: Choose exercises that you enjoy to make the routine more sustainable.

- Workout Buddy: Exercise with a friend or join a fitness group to stay accountable and make workouts more enjoyable. - Variety: Mix up your routine to prevent boredom and keep your workouts interesting.

- Reward System: Set up a reward system for meeting workout goals to keep yourself motivated.

5. Overcoming Common Exercise Barriers
Identifying and overcoming common barriers to exercise can help maintain a consistent workout routine.

Key Points:
- Lack of Time: Schedule workouts as you would any other important activity, break workouts into shorter sessions, or incorporate physical activity into daily tasks.
- Lack of Motivation: Use the tips and strategies for staying motivated, such as setting goals, tracking progress, and finding enjoyable activities.
- Physical Limitations: Modify exercises to fit your abilities, consult a fitness professional for personalized adaptations, and focus on what you can do rather than what you cannot.

Cost: Utilize free or low-cost resources, such as online workout videos, community parks, or home exercise equipment.

- Safety Concerns: Ensure proper warm-up and cool-down, use correct form, and start with lower intensity if you are new to exercise to prevent injuries. By understanding the benefits of exercise, incorporating different types of exercises, designing an effective workout routine, staying motivated, and overcoming common barriers, individuals can achieve their fitness goals and maintain a healthy lifestyle.

# Chapter 3

## Tip 3: Hydration and Sleep

### The Important of Water in Weight Loss

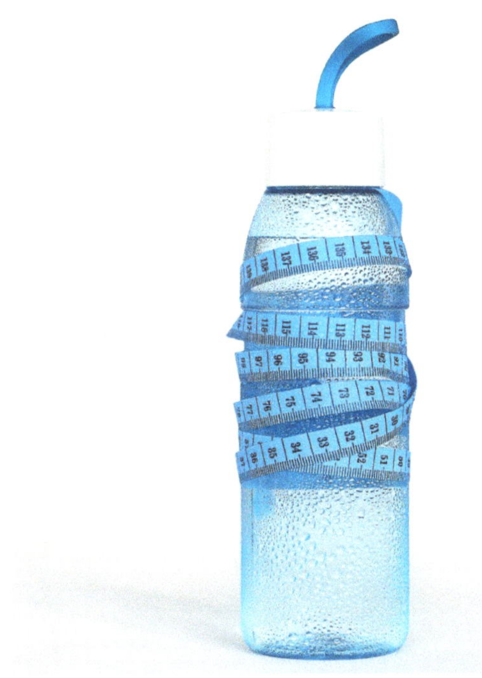

Water is important in weight loss for a variety of reasons:

1. Appetite Suppression: Drinking water before meals might help curb your appetite, making you feel fuller and less inclined to overeat. This is because water occupies space in the stomach, communicating to your brain that you are full.

2. Metabolism Boost: Research has shown that drinking water increases the number of calories expended at rest, often known as resting energy expenditure. Drinking cold water can be especially beneficial because the body expends energy to get the water to body temperature.

3. Calorie-free: Unlike sugary beverages, water contains no calories. Replacing high-calorie beverages with water can drastically reduce total calorie intake.

4. Detoxification: Water improves kidney and liver function, which aids in the removal of toxins from the body. This is critical for sustaining a healthy metabolism.

5. Improved Exercise Performance: Staying hydrated is essential for peak physical performance. Dehydration can cause weariness and decreased motivation, limiting your ability to exercise efficiently and burn calories.

How much water should you drink?

The quantity of water an individual should consume depends on various factors such as age, gender, weight, activity level, and weather. However, general recommendations include:

1. The 8x8 Rule: A frequent guideline is to drink eight 8-ounce glasses of water every day, which equals roughly 2 liters or half a gallon. This is a sensible objective for many people.

2. Body Weight: For a more individualized approach, drink half ounce to one ounce of water for every pound you weigh. For instance, if you weigh 150 pounds, you should drink 75-150 ounces of water every day.

3. Activity Level: If you are active or live in a hot climate, you may require additional water. It's critical to listen to your body and drink extra

when you're thirsty or your urine turns dark yellow.

4. Hydration Indicators: Pay attention to markers of hydration, such as urine color (pale yellow indicates enough hydration) and frequency of urination. Thirst is an obvious but important sign.

The relationship between sleep and weight

Sleep and weight are closely related:

1. Hormonal Balance: Inadequate sleep affects the balance of important hormones that control hunger. Ghrelin, the hormone that promotes appetite, rises, while leptin, the hormone that

indicates fullness, falls. This can cause increased hunger and calorie intake.

2. Metabolism: Inadequate sleep might slow your metabolism. According to studies, sleep deprivation can limit the quantity of calories burned at rest, making weight loss more difficult.

3. Insulin Sensitivity: Sleep deprivation alters the way your body processes insulin, the hormone that regulates blood sugar levels. Insulin resistance can cause elevated blood glucose levels and increased fat storage.

4. Desires and Decision Making: A lack of sleep can impair your brain's ability to make appropriate eating choices while increasing your desire for high-calorie, sugary foods.

5. Energy and Exercise: Lack of sleep can lead to low energy levels, making it more difficult to stay active and keep to a workout plan, which is vital for weight loss.

Tips to Improve Sleep Quality

Improving sleep quality entails building a favorable sleep environment and developing excellent habits:

1. Maintain a consistent schedule: Go to bed and wake up at the same time every day, including weekends. This helps to adjust your brain's internal clock.

2. Create a relaxing bedtime routine that includes calming activities such as reading,

having a warm bath, or practicing relaxation techniques.

3. Sleep Environment: Keep your bedroom dark, cold, and quiet. Consider installing blackout curtains, a white noise machine, or an eye mask.

4. Limit Screen Time: Avoid using screens (phones, tablets, computers) for at least an hour before bedtime. The blue light emitted by these devices can disrupt the production of melatonin, a hormone that governs sleep.

5. Avoid Stimulants: Limit your caffeine and nicotine intake, particularly in the afternoon and evening. These drinks may interfere with your ability to fall asleep.

6. Diet and Exercise: Engaging in regular physical activity and eating a balanced diet will help you sleep better. However, avoid strong exercise close to bedtime.

Dealing With Sleep Disorders

If you feel you have a sleep condition, you should seek professional help. Below are some typical sleep problems and associated treatments:

1. Insomnia refers to difficulty falling or staying asleep. Insomnia treatment methods include cognitive-behavioral therapy (CBT-I), medicines, and lifestyle changes.

2. Sleep Apnea: Interrupted breathing during sleep, frequently accompanied by snoring. CPAP

machines, lifestyle adjustments, and, in certain situations, surgery are all options for treatment.

3. Restless Legs Syndrome (RLS): Uncomfortable sensations in the legs and a need to move them. Medication, lifestyle modifications, and addressing underlying disorders may all be part of the treatment plan.

4. Narcolepsy: Excessive daytime tiredness and unexpected sleep attacks. Medication and lifestyle changes are frequently used to treat the condition.

5. Circadian Rhythm Disorders: Sleep-wake cycle disruptions, including delayed sleep phase syndrome. Light therapy, chronotherapy, and sticking to a regular sleep pattern are all options for treatment.

Understanding and treating hydration and sleep can help you lose weight and improve your overall health. These aspects are sometimes forgotten, yet they are critical to reaching and maintaining a healthy weight.

# Chapter 4

## Tip 4: Mindful Eating

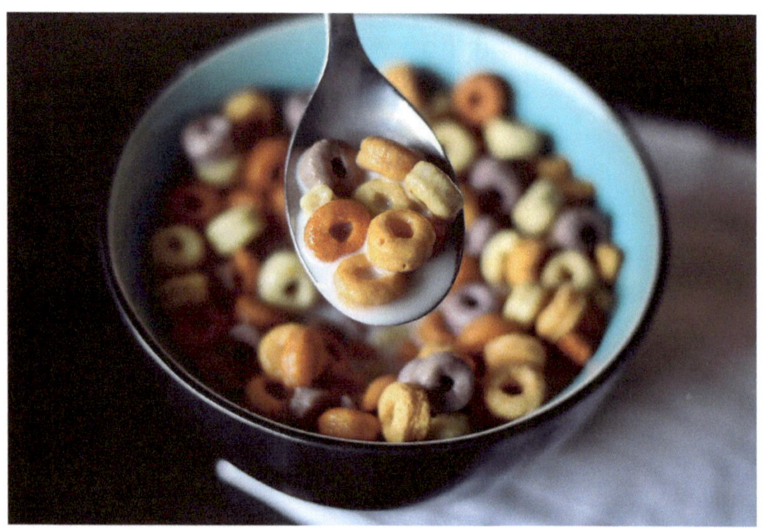

## 1. What is Mindful Eating?

Mindful eating is a practice of being fully present and engaged during meals, focusing on the experience of eating without distraction. It involves paying close attention to the sensations, flavors, and textures of food as well as the body's hunger and fullness signals. Unlike dieting, mindful eating is not about restriction or rules but cultivating a healthy and positive relationship with food.

Key points:

- Being present and attentive throughout meals, paying attention to the sensory experience, and listening to bodily signals for hunger and fullness.

- Developing a pleasant connection with food free of judgment or constraint.

2. Techniques to practice Mindful Eating Several techniques can help individuals practice mindful eating. These techniques encourage slowing down and being present in the moment to enhance the eating experience.

Key Techniques:
-Eat slowly: Take small bites and chew thoroughly, allowing time to savor each mouthful.
- Remove Distractions: Avoid multitasking while eating; turn off the TV, put away your phone, and focus solely on your meal.
- Engage your senses: Pay attention to the colors, scents, textures, and tastes of your meal.

- Pause and Reflect: Take a moment before eating to appreciate the food and the effort that went into preparing it.
- Listen to Your Body: Check in with your hunger and fullness levels before, during, and after meals to eat in response to physical cues rather than emotional ones.

3. Recognizing Hunger and Fullness Cues Understanding and responding to the body's natural hunger and fullness signals is a key aspect of mindful eating. This helps prevent overeating and promotes a balanced approach to food consumption.

Key Points:

- Hunger Cues: Recognize signs of true hunger, such as stomach growling, lightheadedness, or a lack of energy.
- Fullness Cues: Notice signals of satiety, like a comfortably full stomach, decreased interest in food, or a sense of satisfaction.
- Scale of Hunger: Use a hunger scale (from 1 to 10) to gauge your hunger and fullness levels, aiming to eat when moderately hungry and stop when comfortably full.

4. Emotional Eating: Causes and Solutions. Emotional eating happens when people eat to deal with their emotions rather than to meet their hunger. Identifying the reasons for emotional eating and developing alternate coping strategies for mindful eating.

Key Points:

- Common Triggers: Stress, boredom, sadness, or loneliness can often lead to emotional eating.

 - Awareness: Recognize when you are eating in response to emotions rather than physical hunger.

- Alternative Coping Strategies: Instead of using food to control your emotions, it's ideal you engage in exercise, mindfulness or interacting with a friend as this will help improve your mental and physical health.

- Seek professional guidance: Seeking professional guidance from a therapist or counselor. This will go a long way to do away with emotions eating.


5. Creating a Positive Eating Environment The environment in which you eat can significantly impact your eating habits and overall

relationship with food. A positive eating environment promotes relaxation and mindfulness during meals.


Key Points:

- Set the Scene: Create a calm and pleasant atmosphere by setting the table nicely, playing soft music, and minimizing noise and distractions.

 - Mindful Dining: Encourage family or dining companions to engage in conversation and focus on the meal, promoting a sense of connection and enjoyment.

- Meal Preparation: Take time to prepare meals thoughtfully and with care, enhancing the appreciation of the food.

-Enjoy the Process: Treat meals as an opportunity to relax and enjoy the experience of eating, rather than rushing through it.

By implementing these practices, individuals can develop a healthier relationship with food, leading to improved physical and emotional well-being. Mindful eating encourages a balanced approach to nutrition, emphasizing the importance of listening to the body and enjoying the process of eating.

# Chapter 5

## Tip 5 - Stress Management

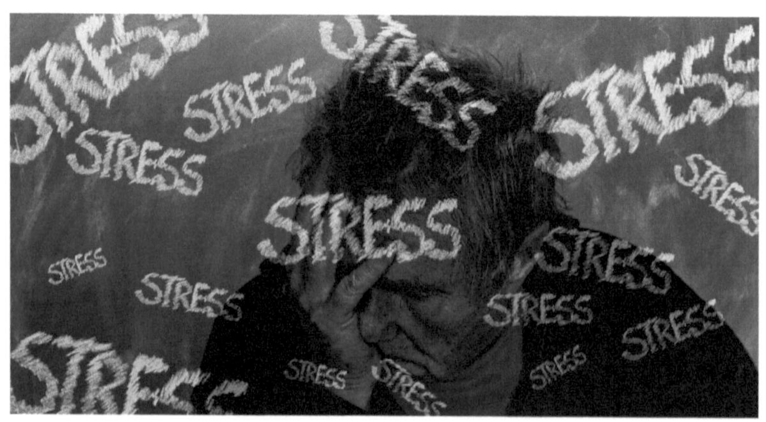


1. Understanding the Impact of Stress on Weight:

- Stress can have a significant impact on weight due to its effects on hormone levels, metabolism, and eating habits.
- Cortisol, the primary stress hormone, can lead to increased appetite and cravings for unhealthy, high-calorie foods. - Chronic stress may disrupt sleep patterns, leading to fatigue and overeating as a coping mechanism.
- Stress-induced eating behaviors can contribute to weight gain and difficulty in weight management.

2. Stress Reduction Techniques: Meditation, Yoga, and More:
- Meditation: This involves focusing the mind and eliminating the stream of jumbled thoughts that may be crowding your mind and causing stress. Regular meditation can reduce stress levels and promote emotional well-being.

- Yoga: Combines physical position, breathing techniques, and meditation or relaxation. It helps in reducing stress, improving flexibility, and enhancing overall health.

- Deep Breathing Exercises: Controlled breathing techniques can activate the body's relaxation response, reducing stress and promoting a sense of calm. - Progressive Muscle Relaxation: Involves tensing and then relaxing each muscle group in the body, promoting physical relaxation and stress relief.

- Mindfulness Practices: Encourage being present in the moment and accepting one's thoughts and feelings without judgment, which can help reduce stress and enhance overall well-being.

3. Creating a Stress-Reduction Plan:

- Identify Stress: Recognize the sources of stress in your life, whether they are related to work, relationships, finances, or health.

- Develop Coping Strategies: Once stressors are identified, create a plan to address them. This may involve utilizing stress reduction techniques such as meditation, exercise, or seeking support from others.

- Time Management: Organize your time effectively to prioritize tasks and reduce feelings of overwhelm and stress.

- Setting Boundaries: Learn to say no to additional commitments or responsibilities when feeling overwhelmed, and establish healthy boundaries to protect your time and energy.

- Self-Care Practices: Engage in activities that promote relaxation and well-being, such as spending time in nature, pursuing hobbies, or practicing gratitude.

4. The Role of Support Systems:
- Friends and Family: Cultivate supportive relationships with friends and family members who can offer understanding, encouragement, and practical assistance during stressful times.
- Support Groups: Joining support groups or seeking professional counseling can provide additional resources and coping strategies for managing stress effectively.
- Communication: Open and honest communication with trusted individuals can help alleviate feelings of isolation and provide opportunities for sharing concerns and seeking advice.

5. Balancing Work, Life, and Health:

- Prioritize Self-Care: Recognize the importance of maintaining a healthy balance between work, personal life, and health. Make time for activities that promote physical and emotional well-being.
- Set Realistic Goals: Establish achievable goals that align with your values and priorities, and break them down into manageable steps to avoid feeling overwhelmed.
- Time Management: Use effective time management techniques to allocate time for work, relaxation, social activities, and self-care.
- Boundaries: Establish clear boundaries between work and personal life to prevent burnout and maintain a healthy work-life balance.
- Flexibility: Be open to adjusting your schedule and priorities as needed to accommodate

unexpected changes and maintain balance in your life.

# Conclusion

In "Weight Loss Guide: 5 Tips to Lose Weight," Dr.    Collins has outlined a comprehensive approach to achieving sustainable weight loss and overall well-being. Throughout the book, the journey to a healthier lifestyle has been meticulously mapped out, focusing on balanced nutrition, regular physical activity, hydration, sleep management, mindful eating, and stress reduction.

By debunking myths surrounding weight loss, setting realistic goals, understanding the significance of balanced nutrition, incorporating regular exercise, staying hydrated, prioritizing quality sleep, practicing mindful eating, and managing stress effectively, individuals can embark on a transformative journey toward a healthier self. The key takeaway from this guide is the holistic nature of weight loss, emphasizing the importance of addressing physical, mental, and emotional health aspects. By adopting the principles outlined in this book, readers can not only achieve their weight loss goals but also cultivate a sustainable and fulfilling lifestyle that promotes long-term well-being. Dr. Hannah Collins's insights serve as a valuable roadmap for anyone seeking to embark on a successful and enduring journey toward a healthier and happier life.

# Recommendation

"Weight Loss Guide: 5 Tips to Lose Weight" by Dr. Hannah Collins is a must-read for anyone seeking a comprehensive approach to achieving sustainable weight loss and overall well-being. Dr. Collins meticulously outlines the journey to a healthier lifestyle, focusing on balanced nutrition, regular physical activity, hydration, sleep management, mindful eating, and stress reduction.

By debunking myths surrounding weight loss, setting realistic goals, understanding the significance of balanced nutrition, incorporating regular exercise, staying hydrated, prioritizing quality sleep, practicing mindful eating, and managing stress effectively, readers can embark on a transformative journey toward a healthier self. This book serves as a valuable roadmap for anyone seeking to achieve their weight loss goals and cultivate a sustainable and fulfilling lifestyle that promotes long-term well-being. Dr. Hannah Collins's insights are both practical and profound, making this guide an indispensable resource for anyone looking to lead a healthier and happier life.